Read a Bit! Talk a Bit! Dog

Written by Gunilla Denton Cook

Published by Denton Cook Pty Ltd
Copyright Denton Cook Pty Ltd 2013
ABN 5403936874
Sydney Australia
Phone +61 2 9651 3558
Fax   +61 2 9651 3007
Email: dentoncook@bigpond.com
Cover photo by Andrew Cook

Read a Bit! Talk a Bit! is a series of reading activity books intended for people with dementia and/or Alzheimer's disease. The books start with a short article for the group to read, followed by a number of questions for the group leader to ask and engage the participants in conversation to encourage personal and meaningful reminiscences to flow.

All the reading pages are in large type, 44 pt, and the text is only on one page per spread in order to help the individual to concentrate on the text and to minimise the constraints of visual impairment.

Memories recalled from earlier in life are often very therapeutic for all and especially for people with memory impairment. These questions are formulated to create meaningful engagement with the past. Remembering increases self esteem and a feeling of positive worth as the participants recall personal experiences.

This series of books successfully achieve this thanks to the range of familiar topics and questions to prompt and encourage discussions.

Titles available:

At the Movies	Lawnmower	Scissors
Cake	Money	Soup
Cat	Pencil	Stamps
Chickens	Perfume	Teddy Bear
Dog	Safety Pin	Telephone
Garden	Sandwich	

Dog is man's best friend, so the saying goes. Dogs have been an important part of our lives for thousands of years.

__Pass to next reader__

We still use dogs for many important jobs. They happily help us to herd sheep and cattle, to find lost people, drugs, and explosives.

Pass to next reader

Read a Bit! Talk a Bit! Dog written by Gunilla Denton Cook.
©2013 Denton Cook Pty Ltd

Larger dogs often enjoy pulling our loads and guarding our homes, farms, and places of work.

Pass to next reader

These days most of us have dogs for pleasure. Having a pet is good for us, the medical profession tells us. It is said to lower our heart rate and to make us feel better in general.

Pass to next reader

Dog owners tend to socialise more with the surroundings. It is also said that one doesn't have to own a dog to draw benefit from it.

Pass to next reader

We are told that it is enough to be around pets to feel better and calmer from their presence.

__Pass to next reader__

There are many different theories as to where the dog originated. Some believe that they go back as far as the dinosaurs.

Pass to next reader

Others are convinced that they stem from an Asian wolf around 80,000 years ago. The theories are many.

Pass to next reader

It is estimated that there are approximately four hundred million dogs in the world today.

Pass to next reader

There are many different breeds, colours and sizes of dogs. The vast majority of them are companion dogs.

Pass to next reader

Who can resist the warm greetings we get when we come home after having been away from them?

Pass to next reader

If we treat our pets with the respect and love they deserve, they will help us remain healthier for longer and enjoy our lives.

__Pass to group leader__

Questions

1. Did you have a pet while you grew up? What kind of pet was it?

2. If you had a dog, what was its name?

3. Do you know what breed of dog it was?

4. What kind of dog is your favourite breed today?

5. Do you prefer small dogs or big dogs?

6. Can you name the different colours dogs come in?
    Black, white, tan, brown, brindle, grey, blue (grey), apricot, etc.

7. How often did you walk your dog?

8. Who fed the dog in your house?

9. What was your dog's favourite food?

10. Did your dog sleep in the house or did it stay outside?

11. What was the naughtiest thing your dog ever did?

12. How often did you play with the dog?

13. How many dogs have you had?

14. Did you have one particular dog that was your favourite?

Read a Bit! Talk a Bit! Dog written by Gunilla Denton Cook.
©2013 Denton Cook Pty Ltd

15. Who did the grooming of your dog?

16. Have you ever tried to clip a dog with scissors? Did the dog look good after your hard work?

17. When you gave your dog a bath, who got the wettest, you or the dog?

18. Did you, or someone you know, use a dog in a professional capacity?

19. How many professions can you think of that use dogs?
    Police, armed forces, security guards, farmers, etc.

20. Did you train your dog to do tricks? What were they?

21. Can you name one dog breed for every letter in the alphabet?

A. *Airedale terrier*
B. *Basset*
C. *Collie, Chow Chow, Cocker Spaniel, Corgi*
D. *Dachshund, Dalmatian, Doberman*
E. *English sheepdog*
F. *Fox terrier*
G. *Great Dane, Greyhound*
H. *Harrier*
I. *Irish wolfhound*
J. *Jack Russell*
K. *King Charles Spaniel*
L. *Labrador*
M. *Maltese*
N. *Newfoundland*
O. *Old English Bulldog*

P.   *Papillion, Pointer, Poodle, Pomeranian, Pug*
Q.
R.   *Rottweiler, Rhodesian Ridgeback*
S.   *Samoyed, Shar Pei*
T.   *Terrier*
U.
V.   *Vizsla*
W.   *Welsh Corgi, Whippet*
X.
Y.   *Yorkshire terrier*
Z.

www.ingramcontent.com/pod-product-compliance
Lightning Source LLC
Chambersburg PA
CBHW081414170526
45166CB00010B/3337